56 Kidney Stone Preventing Juice Recipes:

Juice Your Way to a Healthier and happier life

By

Joe Correa CSN

COPYRIGHT

This publication is designed to provide accurate and authoritative information in regard to the subject matter covered. It is sold with the understanding that neither the author nor the publisher is engaged in rendering medical advice. If medical advice or assistance is needed, consult with a doctor. This book is considered a guide and should not be used in any way detrimental to your health. Consult with a physician before starting this nutritional plan to make sure it's right for you.

ACKNOWLEDGEMENTS

This book is dedicated to my friends and family that have had mild or serious illnesses so that you may find a solution and make the necessary changes in your life.

56 Kidney Stone Preventing Juice Recipes:

Juice Your Way to a Healthier and happier life

By

Joe Correa CSN

CONTENTS

Copyright

Acknowledgements

About The Author

Introduction

56 Kidney Stone Preventing Juice Recipes: Juice Your Way to a Healthier and happier life

Additional Titles from This Author

ABOUT THE AUTHOR

After years of Research, I honestly believe in the positive effects that proper nutrition can have over the body and mind. My knowledge and experience has helped me live healthier throughout the years and which I have shared with family and friends. The more you know about eating and drinking healthier, the sooner you will want to change your life and eating habits.

Nutrition is a key part in the process of being healthy and living longer so get started today. The first step is the most important and the most significant.

INTRODUCTION

56 Kidney Stone Preventing Juice Recipes: Juice Your Way to a Healthier and happier life

By Joe Correa CSN

Kidney Stones are one of the most common urological problems affecting about 14% of the population. Men are mostly affected about three times more often than women. The stone size can vary from small (a couple of millimeters) to a huge one that fits the entire kidney. Most of the time, kidney stones will pass through your urinary tract by themselves. However, sometimes medical treatment is needed to remove a stone that is stuck somewhere along the way.

The formation of kidney stones is directly related to thick urine with little water. This type of urine contains substances that accumulate in the kidney and eventually form the stone. One of the main reasons for thick urine is insufficient fluid intake and a poor diet.

One of the first symptoms of a stone that's growing is severe pain in the back, painful and frequent urination, nausea and vomiting, and blood in the urine.

One of the best ways to prevent the kidney stone formation is a proper diet followed by the right fluid intake, especially freshly squeezed fruit and vegetable juices which are loaded with different antioxidants and other important nutrients.

I have created a wonderful collection of juices that are based on healthy ingredients and will help clean your urinary tract and prevent the stones from forming. You will find some amazing juice recipes with cranberries that are famous for the positive effects they can have on the urinary tract. Cranberries are one of the most common natural cures that doctors prescribe for this condition. Combined with other valuable fruits and vegetables you will find in these recipes, they will stop all the potential infections and boost up your immune system.

Take a couple of minutes every morning and prepare yourself a juice that will help you lead a happy and healthy life!

56 KIDNEY STONE PREVENTING JUICE RECIPES: JUICE YOUR WAY TO A HEALTHIER AND HAPPIER LIFE

1.   Carrot Spinach Juice

Ingredients:

3 large carrots

1 bunch of spinach, torn

1 cup of cauliflower, chopped

1 cup of Swiss chards, torn

¼ tsp of Himalayan salt

2 oz of water

Preparation:

Wash the carrots and chop into thick slices. Set aside.

Combine spinach and Swiss chards in a colander and wash thoroughly under cold running water. Drain, and torn with hands. Set aside.

Trim off the outer leaves of a cauliflower. Wash it and cut into small pieces. Reserve the rest in the refrigerator.

Now, combine carrots, spinach, Swiss chards, and cauliflower in a juicer and process until juiced.

Transfer to serving glasses and stir in the salt and water.

Add few ice cubes and serve immediately.

Nutritional information per serving: Kcal: 138, Protein: 14.4g, Carbs: 39.7g, Fats: 2.2g

2.   Avocado Broccoli Juice

Ingredients:

1 cup of avocado, chopped

1 cup of broccoli, chopped

1 large cucumber

1 large lemon, peeled

1 large lime, peeled

3 oz of water

Preparation:

Peel the avocado and cut in half. Remove the pit and cut into chunks. Set aside.

Wash the broccoli and chop into small pieces. Set aside.

Wash the cucumber and cut in thick slices. Set aside.

Peel the lemon and lime. Cut lengthwise in half. Set aside.

Now, process avocado, broccoli, cucumber, lemon, and lime in a juicer. Transfer to serving glasses and stir in the water.

Add some ice and serve immediately.

Note:

Lemon and lime contain a high amount of citrate, so make sure to add more water than usual.

Nutritional information per serving: Kcal: 281, Protein: 8.3g, Carbs: 38.8g, Fats: 22.8g

3.   Blueberries Watermelon Juice

Ingredients:

2 cups of blueberries

2 cups of watermelon, seeded

1 large grapefruit, chopped

1 tbsp of liquid honey

2 oz of water

Preparation:

Wash the blueberries under cold running water. Drain and set aside.

Cut the watermelon lengthwise. For 2 cups, you will need about 2 large wedges. Peel and cut into chunks. Remove the seeds and set aside. Reserve the rest of the melon for some other juices.

Peel the grapefruit and divide into wedges. Set aside.

Now, process blueberries, watermelon, and grapefruit in a juicer. Transfer to serving glasses and stir in the honey and water.

Refrigerate for 15 minutes before serving.

Enjoy!

Nutritional information per serving: Kcal: 375, Protein: 5.9g, Carbs: 92.1g, Fats: 1.7g

4.   Coconut Mango Juice

Ingredients:

1 large mango, chopped

1 cup of pomegranate seeds

1 large carrot

1 small Granny Smith apple, cored

2 oz of coconut water

Preparation:

Wash the mango and cut into small chunks. Set aside.

Cut the top of the pomegranate fruit using a sharp knife. Slice down to each of the white membranes inside of the fruit. Pop the seeds into a medium bowl.

Wash the carrot and cut into thick slices. Set aside.

Wash the apple and remove the core. Cut into bite-sized pieces and set aside.

Now, combine mango, pomegranate seeds, carrot, and apple in a juicer and process until juiced.

Transfer to serving glasses and stir in the coconut water.

Refrigerate or add some ice and serve immediately.

Nutritional information per serving: Kcal: 338, Protein: 5.5g, Carbs: 94.1g, Fats: 2.7g

5.   Cherry Tomato-Watercress Juice

Ingredients:

1 cup of cherry tomatoes, halved

1 cup of watercress, chopped

1 cup of pumpkin, chopped

1 cup of collard greens, chopped

1 large cucumber

Preparation:

Wash the tomatoes and place them in a bowl. Cut in half and reserve the juice in the bowl while cutting. Set aside.

Combine watercress and collard greens in a colander and wash thoroughly. Torn with hands and set aside.

Peel the pumpkin and cut in half. Scoop out the seeds using a spoon. Cut one large wedge and peel it. Cut into small chunks and set aside. Reserve the rest for later.

Wash the cucumber and cut into thick slices. Set aside.

Now, process tomatoes, watercress, collard greens, pumpkin, and cucumber in a juicer. Transfer to serving glasses and stir in the reserved tomato juice. Add some ice before serving.

Enjoy!

Nutritional information per serving: Kcal: 96, Protein: 6.4g, Carbs: 27.4g, Fats: 1g

6.   Spinach Artichoke Juice

Ingredients:

1 large bunch of spinach

1 large artichoke head

1 cup of sweet potatoes, cubed

1 cup of turnip greens, chopped

1 cup of basil, chopped

2 oz of water

¼ tsp of Himalayan salt

Preparation:

Combine spinach, turnip greens, and basil in a colander and wash under cold running water. Drain and chop it roughly with your hands and set aside.

Trim off the outer leaves of the artichoke using a sharp knife. Cut into bite-sized pieces and set aside.

Peel the sweet potato and cut into chunks. Set aside.

Now, process spinach, turnip greens, basil, artichoke, and sweet potato in a juicer. Transfer to serving glasses and stir in the water and Himalayan salt.

Add some ice and serve immediately.

Nutritional information per serving: Kcal: 202, Protein: 18.6g, Carbs: 60.7g, Fats: 1.9g

7.   Butternut Squash Bean Juice

Ingredients:

1 cup of butternut squash, chopped

1 cup of green beans, chopped

1 cup fresh celery, torn

1 cup of purple cabbage, torn

1 large cucumber

1 large green bell pepper, seeded

¼ tsp of Himalayan salt

2 oz of water

Preparation:

Peel the butternut squash and remove the seeds using a spoon. Cut into small cubes and reserve the rest of the squash for some other recipe. Wrap in a plastic foil and refrigerate.

Combine purple cabbage and celery in a colander and wash under cold running water. Drain and torn with hands. Set aside.

Wash the green beans cut into bite-sized pieces. Set aside.

Wash the cucumber and cut into thick slices. Set aside.

Wash the bell pepper and cut in half. Remove the seeds and chop into small pieces. Set aside.

Now, process butternut squash, cabbage, celery, green beans, cucumber, and bell pepper in a juicer.

Transfer to serving glasses and stir in the salt and water. Refrigerate for 30 minutes before serving.

Enjoy!

Nutritional information per serving: Kcal: 163, Protein: 7.7g, Carbs: 48.2g, Fats: 1.1g

8.　Kiwi Carrot Juice

Ingredients:

2 large kiwis, peeled

2 large carrots

1 large Honeycrisp apple, cored

1 cup of mint, chopped

1 large orange, peeled

2 oz of water

Preparation:

Peel the kiwis and cut lengthwise in half. Set aside.

Wash the carrots and cut into thick slices. Set aside

Wash the apple and remove the core. Cut into bite-sized pieces and set aside.

Wash the fresh mint and roughly chop it. Set aside.

Now, combine kiwis, carrots, apple, and mint in a juicer and process until juiced. Transfer to serving glasses and add some ice before serving.

Enjoy!

Nutritional information per serving: Kcal: 292, Protein: 6.1g, Carbs: 88.6g, Fats: 1.8g

9.   Bloody Beets Juice

Ingredients:

2 large beets, trimmed

1 large red apple, cored

1 cup of pomegranate seeds

1 large cucumber

1 small ginger knob, 1-inch

Preparation:

Wash the beets and trim off the green parts. Cut into small pieces and set aside.

Wash the apple and remove the core. Cut into bite-sized pieces and set aside.

Cut the top of the pomegranate fruit using a sharp knife. Slice down to each of the white membranes inside of the fruit. Pop the seeds into a medium bowl.

Wash the cucumber and cut into thick slices. Set aside.

Peel the ginger knob and set aside.

Now, process beets, apple, pomegranate seeds, cucumber and ginger knob in a juicer. Transfer to serving glasses and add some ice. You can stir in one tablespoon of honey, but this is optional.

Serve immediately.

Nutritional information per serving: Kcal: 285, Protein: 8g, Carbs: 81.6g, Fats: 2.2g

10.   Carrot Grape Juice

Ingredients:

3 large carrots

1 cup of green grapes

1 Granny Smith apple, cored

1 large lemon, peeled

A handful of spinach

2 oz of water

Preparation:

Wash the carrots and cut into thick slices. Set aside.

Wash the grapes and set aside.

Wash the apple and remove the core. Cut into bite-sized pieces and set aside.

Peel the lemon and cut lengthwise in half. Set aside.

Wash the spinach thoroughly under cold running water. Roughly chop it and set aside.

Now, combine carrots, grapes, apple, lemon, and spinach in a juicer and process until juiced. Transfer to serving glasses and stir in the water.

Refrigerate for 20 minutes before serving.

Enjoy!

Nutritional information per serving: Kcal: 208, Protein: 1.4g, Carbs: 62.6g, Fats: 1.4g

11.   Green Crookneck Juice

Ingredients:

1 cup of crookneck squash

1 cup of collard greens, torn

1 cup of kale, torn

1 cup Romaine lettuce, torn

1 large cucumber

½ tsp of Himalayan salt

¼ tsp of Cayenne pepper, ground

2 oz of water

Preparation:

Wash the crookneck squash and cut in half. Scoop out the seeds using a spoon. Cut into small chunks and set aside. Reserve the rest for another juice.

Combine collard greens, kale, and lettuce in a colander. Wash thoroughly under cold running water and torn with hands. Set aside.

Wash the cucumber and chop into thick slices. Set aside.

Now, combine crookneck squash, collard greens, kale, lettuce, and cucumber in a juicer and process until juiced.

Transfer to serving glasses and stir in the salt, Cayenne pepper, and water. Refrigerate for 15 minutes before serving.

Nutritional information per serving: Kcal: 91, Protein: 7.8g, Carbs: 25.2g, Fats: 1.6g

12.   Honeydew Cherry Juice

Ingredients:

1 large honeydew melon wedge

1 cup of fresh cherries

1 large lime, peeled

1 large orange, peeled

1 tbsp of honey, raw

2 oz of coconut water

Preparation:

Cut the honeydew melon lengthwise in half. Scoop out the seeds using a spoon. Cut the large wedges and peel them. Cut into small chunks and place in a bowl. Wrap the rest of the melon in a plastic foil and refrigerate.

Wash the cherries and cut in half. Remove the pits and set aside.

Peel the lime and cut lengthwise in half. Set aside.

Peel the orange and divide into wedges. Set aside.

Now, process honeydew melon, cherries, lime, and orange in a juicer. Transfer to serving glasses and stir in the honey and coconut water.

Add some ice and serve immediately.

Nutritional information per serving: Kcal: 276, Protein: 4.2g, Carbs: 78.9g, Fats: 0.7g

13.   Brussels Sprout Fennel Juice

Ingredients:

2 cups of Brussels sprouts

2 cups of fennel

1 cup of purple cabbage, torn

1 large lemon, peeled

1 cup of beet greens, torn

1 large cucumber

Preparation:

Wash the Brussels sprouts and trim off the outer leaves. Cut in half and set aside.

Wash the fennel bulb and trim off the wilted outer layers. Cut into small chunks and set aside.

Combine cabbage and beet greens in a colander and wash under cold running water. Torn with hands and set aside.

Wash the cucumber and cut into thick slices. Set aside.

Now, combine Brussels sprouts, fennel, cabbage, beet greens, and cucumber in a juicer and process until juiced.

Transfer to serving glasses and add few ice cubes before serving.

Enjoy!

Nutritional information per serving: Kcal: 154, Protein: 12.8g, Carbs: 53g, Fats: 1.5g

14. Orange Mango Juice

Ingredients:

1 cup of mango chunks

1 large orange, peeled

1 large green apple, cored

1 large lime, peeled

1 small ginger root knob, 1-inch

2 oz of water

Preparation:

Wash the mango and cut into chunks. Fill the measuring cup and refrigerate the rest for some other juice.

Peel the orange and divide into wedges. Set aside.

Wash the apple and remove the core. Cut into bite-sized pieces and set aside.

Peel the lime and cut lengthwise in half. Set aside.

Peel the ginger knob and set aside.

Now, process mango, orange, apple, lime, and ginger in a juicer. Transfer to serving glasses and stir in the water.

Add some ice and serve immediately.

Enjoy!

Nutritional information per serving: Kcal: 268, Protein: 12.8g, Carbs: 53g, Fats: 1.5g

15.   Zucchini Pepper Juice

Ingredients:

2 large yellow bell peppers, chopped

1 large zucchini, chopped

1cup of watercress, torn

1 large carrot

1 cup of parsnips, chopped

½ tsp of Himalayan salt

Preparation:

Wash the bell peppers and cut in half. Remove the seeds and chop into small pieces. Set aside.

Peel the zucchini and cut in half. Scoop out the seeds and cut into small chunks. Set aside.

Wash the watercress thoroughly under cold running water and torn with hands. Set aside.

Wash the carrot and parsnips. Cut into bite-sized pieces and set aside.

Now, process bell peppers, zucchini, watercress, carrot, and parsnips in a juicer. Transfer to serving glasses and stir in the salt.

Refrigerate for 15 minutes before serving.

Nutritional information per serving: Kcal: 243, Protein: 11.2g, Carbs: 70g, Fats: 2.5g

16.   Asparagus Celery Juice

Ingredients:

1 cup of asparagus, trimmed

1 cup of celery, chopped

1 cup of fresh kale, torn

1 cup of mustard greens, torn

1 large lemon

1 large cucumber

Preparation:

Wash the asparagus and trim off the woody ends. Cut into small pieces and set aside.

Wash the celery thoroughly and cut into bite-sized pieces. Set aside.

Combine kale and mustard greens in a colander and wash under cold running water. Torn with hands and set aside.

Peel the lemon and cut lengthwise in half. Set aside.

Wash the cucumber and cut into thick slices. Set aside.

Now, process asparagus, celery, kale, mustard greens, lemon, and cucumber in a juicer.

Transfer to serving glasses and add few ice cubes before serving.

Enjoy!

Nutritional information per serving: Kcal: 107, Protein: 10.7g, Carbs: 33g, Fats: 1.7g

17.   Raspberry Mint Juice

Ingredients:

2 cups of fresh raspberries

2 cups of fresh mint, torn

1 large orange

1 large green apple, cored

1 large lime

2 oz of water

Preparation:

Wash the raspberries under cold running water and set aside.

Wash the mint thoroughly and torn with hands. Set aside.

Peel the orange and divide into wedges. Set aside.

Peel the apple and remove the core. Cut into bite-sized pieces and set aside.

Peel the lime and cut lengthwise in half. Set aside.

Now, process raspberries, mint, orange, apple, and lime in a juicer. Transfer to serving glasses and stir in the water.

Add some ice and serve immediately.

Nutritional information per serving: Kcal: 258, Protein: 7.6g, Carbs: 90.1g, Fats: 2.7g

18.   Tomato Pumpkin Juice

Ingredients:

1 cup of pumpkin, cubed

2 medium-sized Roma tomatoes, chopped

1 cup of fresh basil, torn

1 large cucumber

¼ tsp of dried oregano

½ tsp of sea salt

2 oz of water

Preparation:

Peel the pumpkin and cut in half. Scoop out the seeds using a spoon. Cut one large wedge and peel it. Cut into small chunks and set aside. Reserve the rest for later.

Wash the tomatoes and place them in a bowl. Cut into quarters and reserve the juice while cutting. Set aside.

Wash the basil thoroughly under cold running water. Torn with hands and set aside.

Wash the cucumber and cut into thick slices. Set aside.

Now, process pumpkin, tomatoes, basil, and cucumber in a juicer. Transfer to serving glasses and stir in the oregano, salt, water, and reserved tomato juice.

Refrigerate for 10 minutes before serving.

Enjoy!

Nutritional information per serving: Kcal: 87, Protein: 4.9g, Carbs: 23.9g, Fats: 0.9g

19.   Blackberry Peach Juice

Ingredients:

1 cup of fresh blackberries

2 medium-sized peaches

1 large lemon

1 cup of cantaloupe, cubed

1 large carrot

1 small yellow apple, cored

2 oz of water

Preparation:

Wash the blackberries under cold running water and set aside.

Wash the peaches and cut in half. Remove the pits and cut into bite-sized pieces. Set aside.

Cut the cantaloupe in half. Scoop out the seeds and flesh. Cut two wedges and peel them. Chop into chunks and set aside. Reserve the rest of the cantaloupe in a refrigerator.

Wash the carrot and cut into thick slices. Set aside.

Wash the apple and remove the core. Cut into bite-sized pieces and set aside.

Now, process blackberries, peaches, cantaloupe, carrot, and apple in a juicer. Transfer to serving glasses and stir in the water.

Add some ice cubes and serve immediately.

Nutritional information per serving: Kcal: 272, Protein: 7.7g, Carbs: 85g, Fats: 2.3g

20. Artichoke Zucchini Juice

Ingredients:

1 large artichoke

1 medium-sized zucchini

1 large carrot

1 red leaf lettuce, torn

1 cup of watercress, torn

3 oz of water

Preparation:

Trim off the outer leaves of the artichoke using a sharp knife. Cut into small pieces and set aside.

Peel the zucchini and cut in half. Scoop out the seeds and cut into chunks. Set aside. Set aside.

Wash the carrot and cut into thick slices. Set aside.

Combine red leaf lettuce and watercress in a colander. Wash under cold running water. Drain and torn with hands. Set aside.

Now, process artichoke, zucchini, carrot, red leaf lettuce, and watercress in a juicer. Transfer to serving glasses and stir in the water.

You can sprinkle with some fresh mint, but this is optional.

Add few ice cubes and serve immediately.

Nutritional information per serving: Kcal: 94, Protein: 9.4g, Carbs: 31.1g, Fats: 1.1g

21.　Orange Pomegranate Juice

Ingredients:

1 large orange

1 cup of pomegranate seeds

1 cup of purple cabbage, torn

1 cup of sweet potatoes, cubed

1 large cucumber

2 oz of water

Preparation:

Peel the orange and divide into wedges. Set aside.

Cut the top of the pomegranate fruit using a sharp knife. Slice down to each of the white membranes inside of the fruit. Pop the seeds into a measuring cup and set aside.

Wash the cabbage thoroughly under cold running water. Drain and torn with hands. Set aside.

Peel the sweet potato and cut into cubes. Fill the measuring cup and reserve the rest for another juice. Set aside.

Wash the cucumber and cut into thick slices. Set aside.

Now, combine orange, pomegranate seeds, purple cabbage, sweet potatoes, and cucumber in a juicer and process until juiced.

Transfer to serving glasses and stir in the water. Add some ice cubes and serve immediately.

Enjoy!

Nutritional information per serving: Kcal: 251, Protein: 6.8g, Carbs: 73.1g, Fats: 1.5g

22.   Celery Grapefruit Juice

Ingredients:

2 cups of celery, chopped

2 large grapefruits

1 large lime

2 large carrots

1 ginger root slice, 1-inch

2 oz of water

Preparation:

Wash the celery and chop into small pieces. About 2 large stalks will be enough. Set aside.

Peel the grapefruits and divide into wedges. Set aside.

Peel the lime lengthwise in half. Set aside.

Wash the carrots and cut into thick slices. Set aside.

Peel the ginger slice and set aside.

Now, process celery, grapefruits, lime, carrots, and ginger in a juicer. Transfer to serving glasses and stir in the water.

Refrigerate for 15 minutes before serving.

Enjoy!

Nutritional information per serving: Kcal: 250, Protein: 6.7g, Carbs: 76.3g, Fats: 1.4g

23.   Papaya Cantaloupe Juice

Ingredients:

1 cup of papaya, chopped

1 large green apple, cored

1 cup of cantaloupe, cubed

1 large cucumber

1 large lemon

Preparation:

Peel the papaya and cut lengthwise in half. Scoop out the black seeds and flesh using a spoon. Cut into small chunks and fill the measuring cup. Refrigerate the rest for some other juice recipe. Set aside.

Wash the apple and remove the core. Cut into bite-sized pieces and set aside.

Cut the cantaloupe in half. Scoop out the seeds and flesh. Cut two wedges and peel them. Chop into chunks and set aside. Reserve the rest of the cantaloupe in a refrigerator.

Wash the cucumber and cut into thick slices. Set aside.

Peel the lime and cut lengthwise in half. Set aside.

Now, process papaya, apple, cantaloupe, cucumber, and lime in a juicer. Transfer to serving glasses and add few ice cubes before serving.

Enjoy!

Nutritional information per serving: Kcal: 245, Protein: 5.5g, Carbs: 72.8g, Fats: 1.6g

24.   Guava Squash Juice

Ingredients:

1 cup of butternut squash, chopped

1 large guava

1 large carrot

1 large cucumber

1 large orange

1 tbsp of honey

Preparation:

Peel the butternut squash and remove the seeds using a spoon. Cut into small cubes and reserve the rest of the squash for some other recipe. Wrap in a plastic foil and refrigerate.

Peel the guava and cut into chunks. Set aside.

Wash the carrot and cucumber and cut into thick slices. Set aside.

Now, combine butternut squash, guava, carrot, and cucumber in a juicer and process until juiced.

Transfer to serving glasses and stir in the honey.

Add some ice and serve immediately.

Nutritional information per serving: Kcal: 266, Protein: 7.2g, Carbs: 80.7g, Fats: 1.4g

25.   Blueberry Melon Juice

Ingredients:

1 cup of fresh blueberries

2 cups of watermelon, cubed

1 large Granny Smith's apple

1 cup of Romaine lettuce, torn

3 oz of coconut water

Preparation:

Wash the blueberries under cold running water. Drain and set aside.

Cut the watermelon lengthwise. For one cup, you will need about one large wedge. Peel and cut into chunks. Remove the seeds and set aside. Reserve the rest of the melon for some other juices.

Wash the lettuce thoroughly and torn with hands. Set aside.

Now, combine blueberries, watermelon, apple, and lettuce in a juicer and process until juiced. Transfer to serving glasses and stir in the coconut water.

Add few ice cubes and serve immediately.

Nutritional information per serving: Kcal: 282, Protein: 4.4g, Carbs: 77g, Fats: 1.4g

26.   Lemon Basil Juice

Ingredients:

2 large lemons

2 cups of fresh basil, torn

1 medium-sized orange

1 large cucumber

1 small ginger knob, 1-inch

2 oz of water

Preparation:

Peel the lemons and cut lengthwise in half. Set aside.

Wash the basil leave thoroughly under cold running water. Drain and set aside.

Peel the orange and divide into wedges. Set aside.

Wash the cucumber and cut into thick slices. Set aside.

Peel the ginger root knob and set aside.

Now, combine lemons, basil, orange, cucumber, and ginger in a juicer and process until juiced.

Transfer to serving glasses and stir in the water.

Refrigerate for 20 minutes before serving, or add some ice and serve immediately.

Enjoy!

Note:

Lemon contains a high amount of citrate, so make sure to add more water than usual.

Nutritional information per serving: Kcal: 124, Protein: 6.1g, Carbs: 39.5g, Fats: 1.1g

27.　Swiss Chard Carrot Juice

Ingredients:

3 large carrots

2 cups of Swiss chard

1 cup of cauliflower

1 large lime

1 large orange

2 oz of water

Preparation:

Wash the carrots and cut into thick slices. Set aside.

Wash the Swiss chard thoroughly and torn with hands. Set aside.

Trim off the outer leaves of cauliflower. Wash it and cut into small pieces. Fill the measuring cup and reserve the rest in the refrigerator.

Peel the lime and cut lengthwise in half. Set aside.

Peel the orange and divide into wedges. Set aside.

Now, process carrots, Swiss chard, cauliflower, lime, and orange in a juicer. Transfer to serving glasses and stir in the water.

Add some ice and serve immediately.

Enjoy!

Nutritional information per serving: Kcal: 173, Protein: 7.3g, Carbs: 54g, Fats: 1.2g

28. Red Bell Pepper Beet Juice

Ingredients:

3 large beets, trimmed

2 large red bell peppers, chopped

1 cup of fresh basil

1 large lime

1 cup of red leaf lettuce, torn

1 large cucumber

Preparation:

Wash the beets and trim off the green parts. Cut into small pieces and set aside.

Wash the red bell peppers and cut in half. Remove the seeds and roughly chop it. Set aside.

Peel the lime and cut lengthwise in half. Set aside.

Place the red leaf lettuce in a colander and wash thoroughly under cold running water. Drain and torn with hands. Set aside.

Wash the cucumber and cut into thick slices. Set aside.

Now, process beets, red bell peppers, lime, red leaf lettuce, and cucumber in a juicer. Transfer to serving glasses and add few ice cubes.

Serve immediately.

Nutritional information per serving: Kcal: 208, Protein: 10.5g, Carbs: 59.2g, Fats: 1.9g

29.   Kiwi Kale Juice

Ingredients:

3 large kiwis

1 cup of fresh kale

1 large lemon

1 large green apple, cored

1 cup of fresh mint

A handful of fresh spinach

3 oz of water

Preparation:

Peel the kiwis and lemon. Cut lengthwise in half and set aside.

Wash kale, mint, and spinach and combine in a large bowl. Pour hot water enough to cover the ingredients. Let it soak for 10 minutes. Drain and torn with hands. Set aside.

Wash the apple and remove the core. Cut into bite-sized pieces and set aside.

Now, process kiwis, lemon, kale, mint, spinach, and apple in a juicer. Transfer to serving glasses and stir in the water.

Add some ice and serve immediately.

Enjoy!

Nutritional information per serving: Kcal: 246, Protein: 8.6g, Carbs: 74.5g, Fats: 2.6g

30. Leek Radish Juice

Ingredients:

2 large leeks, chopped

3 large radishes, chopped

2 cups of beet greens, torn

1 cup of collard greens, torn

1 large cucumber

½ tsp of Himalayan salt

¼ tsp of Cayenne pepper, ground

3 oz of water

Preparation:

Wash the leeks and chop into small pieces. Set aside.

Wash the radishes and trim off the green parts. Cut in half and set aside.

Combine beet greens and collard greens in a colander. Wash thoroughly under cold running water. Drain and set aside.

Wash the cucumber and cut into thick slices. Set aside-

Now, combine leeks, radishes, beet greens, collard greens, and cucumber in a juicer and process until juiced.

Transfer to serving glasses and stir in the salt, Cayenne pepper, and water.

Refrigerate for 15 minutes before serving.

Enjoy!

Nutritional information per serving: Kcal: 148, Protein: 7.6g, Carbs: 42.3g, Fats: 1.2g

31.   Fuji Cranberry Juice

Ingredients:

1 cup of cranberries

1 large orange

1 cup of watermelon, cubed

1 small Fuji apple, cored

1 small ginger knob, 1-inch

2 oz of coconut water

Preparation:

Place the cranberries in a colander and wash under cold running water. Drain and set aside.

Peel the orange and divide into wedges. Set aside.

Cut the watermelon lengthwise. For one cup, you will need about 1 large wedge. Peel and cut into chunks. Remove the seeds and set aside. Reserve the rest of the melon for some other juices.

Wash the apple and remove the core. Cut into bite-sized pieces and set aside.

Peel the ginger root knob and set aside.

Now, combine cranberries, orange, watermelon, apple, and ginger in a juicer and process until juiced.

Transfer to serving glasses and stir in the coconut water. Add some ice and serve immediately.

Enjoy!

Nutritional information per serving: Kcal: 223, Protein: 3.8g, Carbs: 66g, Fats: 0.9g

32.   Avocado Pineapple Juice

Ingredients:

1 cup of avocado, cubed

1 cup of pineapple chunks

1 large orange

1 large cucumber

2 oz of water

Preparation:

Peel the avocado and cut in half. Remove the pit and cut into small cubes. Set aside.

Cut the top of a pineapple and peel it using a sharp knife. Cut into small chunks. Reserve the rest of the pineapple in a refrigerator.

Peel the orange and divide into wedges. Set aside.

Wash the cucumber and cut into thick slices. Set aside.

Now, combine avocado, pineapple, orange, and cucumber in a juicer and process until juiced.

Transfer to serving glasses and stir in the water. Add few ice cubes and serve immediately.

Nutritional information per serving: Kcal: 375, Protein: 7.5g, Carbs: 66.6g, Fats: 22.15g

33.　　Agave Plum Juice

Ingredients:

5 large plums, pitted

1 large Granny Smith apple, cored

1 cup of watermelon, diced

1 tbsp of agave nectar

3 oz of water

Preparation:

Wash the plums and cut in half. Remove the pits and cut into small pieces. Set aside.

Wash the apple and remove the core. Cut into bite-sized pieces and set aside.

Cut the watermelon lengthwise. For one cup, you will need about 1 large wedge. Peel and cut into chunks. Remove the seeds and set aside. Reserve the rest of the melon for some other juices.

Now, combine plums, apple, and watermelon in a juicer and blend until juiced.

Transfer to serving glasses and stir in the agave nectar and water. Add some ice and serve.

Enjoy!

Nutritional information per serving: Kcal: 330, Protein: 4.1g, Carbs: 93.2g, Fats: 1.5g

34.   Cauliflower Beet Juice

Ingredients:

1 small cauliflower head, chopped

2 large beets, trimmed

1 large lime

2 large radishes, chopped

¼ tsp of Himalayan salt

3 oz of water

Preparation:

Trim off the outer leaves of cauliflower. Wash it and cut into small pieces. Set aside.

Wash the beets and radishes. Trim off the green parts and cut into bite-sized pieces. Set aside.

Peel the lime and cut lengthwise in half. Set aside.

Now, combine cauliflower, beets, radishes, and lime in a juicer. Transfer to serving glasses and stir in the Himalayan salt and water.

Add some ice cubes and serve immediately.

Nutritional information per serving: Kcal: 135, Protein: 9.3g, Carbs: 41g, Fats: 1.2g

35.   Green Beans Carrot Juice

Ingredients:

1 cup of green beans

3 large carrots

1 large lemon

1 cup of fresh kale, torn

1 large cucumber

1 tbsp of honey, raw

Preparation:

Wash the green beans and place them in a medium pot. Add water enough to cover and soak for at least 2 hours. Set aside.

Wash the carrots and cut into thick slices. Set aside.

Wash the kale thoroughly under cold running water. Drain and set aside.

Now, process green beans, carrots, lemon, kale, and cucumber in a juicer.

Transfer to serving glasses and stir in the honey. Refrigerate for 30 minutes and serve.

Enjoy!

Nutritional information per serving: Kcal: 239, Protein: 9.4g, Carbs: 50g, Fats: 1.8g

36.　Brussels Sprout Cabbage Juice

Ingredients:

2 cups of Brussels sprouts, halved

1 cup of green cabbage, torn

1 large zucchini, chopped

1 cup of celery, chopped

¼ tsp of Himalayan salt

2 oz of water

Preparation:

Wash the Brussels sprouts and trim off the outer leaves. Cut in half and set aside.

Wash the cabbage thoroughly under cold running water. Drain and torn with hands. Set aside.

Peel the zucchini and cut in half. Scoop out the seeds and chop into small pieces. Set aside.

Wash the celery and cut into small pieces. Set aside.

Now, combine Brussels sprouts, cabbage, zucchini, and celery in a juicer and process until juiced. Transfer to serving glasses and stir in the Himalayan salt and water.

Add few ice cubes or refrigerate before serving.

Enjoy!

Nutritional information per serving: Kcal: 115, Protein: 11.7g, Carbs: 33.9g, Fats: 1.8g

37.   Mixed Squash Juice

Ingredients:

1 cup of butternut squash, chopped

1 cup of crookneck squash, chopped

1 large zucchini

1 cup of pumpkin, chopped

1 large carrot

¼ tsp of Himalayan salt

2 oz of water

Preparation:

Peel the butternut squash and remove the seeds using a spoon. Cut into small cubes and reserve the rest of the squash for some other recipe. Wrap in a plastic foil and refrigerate.

Wash the crookneck squash and cut in half. Scoop out the seeds using a spoon. Cut into small chunks and set aside. Reserve the rest for another juice.

Peel the zucchini and cut in lengthwise in half. Scrap out the seeds and cut into chunks. Set aside.

Peel the pumpkin and cut in half. Scoop out the seeds using a spoon. Cut one large wedge and peel it. Cut into small chunks and set aside. Reserve the rest for later.

Wash the carrot and cut into thick slices. Set aside.

Now, process butternut squash, crookneck squash, zucchini, pumpkin, and carrot in a juicer.

Transfer to serving glasses and stir in the Himalayan salt and water. Refrigerate for 15 minutes before serving.

Enjoy!

Nutritional information per serving: Kcal: 163, Protein: 8.4g, Carbs: 45.8g, Fats: 1.8g

38. Blackberry Cantaloupe Juice

Ingredients:

2 cups of blackberries

1 cup of cantaloupe, diced

1 large orange

1 large lemon

1 small Granny Smith apple

Preparation:

Place the blackberries in a colander and wash under cold running water. Drain and set aside.

Cut the cantaloupe in half. Scoop out the seeds and flesh. Cut two wedges and peel them. Chop into chunks and set aside. Reserve the rest of the cantaloupe in a refrigerator.

Peel the orange and divide into wedges. Set aside.

Peel the lemon and cut lengthwise in half. Set aside.

Wash the apple and remove the core. Cut into bite-sized pieces and set aside.

Now, combine blackberries, cantaloupe, orange, lemon, and apple in a juicer and process until juiced. Transfer to serving glasses and refrigerate for 10 minutes before serving.

Enjoy!

Nutritional information per serving: Kcal: 258, Protein: 8.3g, Carbs: 87g, Fats: 2.4g

39.   Peach Apple Juice

Ingredients:

2 large peaches, chopped

1 medium-sized red apple, cored

1 large orange

1 ginger root knob, 1-inch

2 oz of water

Preparation:

Wash the peaches and cut in half. Remove the pits and cut into small pieces. Set aside.

Wash the apple and remove the core. Cut into bite-sized pieces and set aside.

Peel the orange and divide into wedges. Set aside.

Peel the ginger root knob and set aside.

Now, process peaches, apple, orange, and ginger in a juicer. Transfer to serving glasses and stir in the water.

Add some ice or refrigerate before serving.

Nutritional information per serving: Kcal: 294, Protein: 5.6g, Carbs: 85.8g, Fats: 1.5g

40.   Carrot Watermelon Juice

Ingredients:

3 large carrots

1 large green apple, cored

1 large orange

1 cup of watermelon, diced

1 cup of green grapes

1 small ginger root knob, 1-inch

Preparation:

Wash the carrots and cut into thick slices. Set aside.

Wash the apple and remove the core. Cut into bite-sized pieces and set aside.

Peel the orange and divide into wedges. Set aside.

Cut the watermelon lengthwise. For one cup, you will need about 1 large wedge. Peel and cut into chunks. Remove the seeds and set aside. Reserve the rest of the melon for some other juices.

Wash the grapes under cold running water. Drain and set aside.

Peel the ginger root knob and set aside.

Now, combine carrots, apple, orange, watermelon, grapes, and ginger in a juicer and process until juiced.

Transfer to serving glasses and add some ice before serving.

Enjoy!

Nutritional information per serving: Kcal: 335, Protein: 6.2g, Carbs: 98g, Fats: 1.7g

41.   Broccoli Arugula Juice

Ingredients:

1 cup of broccoli

1 cup of arugula, torn

2 large leeks, chopped

1 cup of beet greens, torn

1 cup of collard greens, torn

1 large cucumber

1 large lime

A handful of spinach, torn

Preparation:

Combine arugula, beet greens, collard greens, and spinach in a colander. Wash under cold running water and torn with hands.

Wash the broccoli and cut into small chunks. Set aside.

Wash the leeks and cut into small pieces. Set aside.

Wash the cucumber and cut into thick slices. Set aside.

Peel the lime and cut lengthwise in half. Set aside.

Now, process arugula, beet greens, collard greens, spinach, leeks, broccoli, cucumber, and lime in a juicer. Transfer to serving glasses and refrigerate for 30 minutes before serving.

Enjoy!

Nutritional information per serving: Kcal: 194, Protein: 13.1g, Carbs: 55.7g, Fats: 1.8g

42.   Cranberry Mango Juice

Ingredients:

1 cup of cranberries

1 cup of mango chunks

1 medium-sized green apple, cored

1 large honeydew melon wedge, chopped

1 cup of fresh mint

½ cup of hot water

Preparation:

Place the cranberries in a colander and wash under cold running water. Drain and set aside.

Peel the mango and cut into chunks. Set aside.

Wash the apple and remove the core. Cut into bite-sized pieces and set aside.

Cut the honeydew melon lengthwise in half. Scoop out the seeds using a spoon. Cut the large wedges and peel them. Cut into small chunks and place in a bowl. Wrap the rest of the melon in a plastic foil and refrigerate.

Combine mint with hot water and let it stand for 15 minutes.

Now, process mango, apple, honeydew melon, and mint in a juicer. Transfer to serving glasses and add water from the soaked mint. Refrigerate for 30 minutes before serving.

Nutritional information per serving: Kcal: 261, Protein: 4.3g, Carbs: 79.1g, Fats: 1.5g

43.   Celery Avocado Juice

Ingredients:

3 cups of celery, chopped

1 cup of avocado chunks

1 cup of cantaloupe, chopped

1 cup of fresh basil, torn

1 cup of cucumber, sliced

2 oz of water

Preparation:

Wash the celery and cut into small pieces. Set aside.

Peel the avocado and cut in half. Remove the pit and cut into chunks. Fill the measuring cup and refrigerate the rest for some other juice.

Cut the cantaloupe in half. Scoop out the seeds and flesh. Cut two wedges and peel them. Chop into chunks and set aside. Reserve the rest of the cantaloupe in a refrigerator.

Wash the basil thoroughly under cold running water. Drain and torn with hands. Set aside.

Wash the cucumber and cut into thick slices. Set aside.

Now, process celery, avocado, cantaloupe, basil, and cucumber in a juicer. Transfer to serving glasses and refrigerate for 15 minutes before serving.

Enjoy!

Nutritional information per serving: Kcal: 288, Protein: 7.5g, Carbs: 37.1g, Fats: 23g

44. Grapefruit Raspberry Juice

Ingredients:

1 large grapefruit

1 cup of raspberries

1 large lemon

1 large lime

1 medium-sized yellow apple, cored

4 oz of coconut water

Preparation:

Peel the grapefruit and divide into wedges. Set aside.

Place the raspberries in a colander and wash under cold running water. Drain and set aside.

Peel the lemon and lime. Cut lengthwise in half and set aside.

Wash the apple and remove the core. Cut into bite-sized pieces and set aside.

Now combine grapefruit, raspberries, lemon, lime, and apple in a juicer and process until juiced. Transfer to serving glasses and stir in the coconut water.

Add some ice and serve immediately.

Note:

Lemon and lime contain a high amount of citrate, so make sure to add more water than usual.

Nutritional information per serving: Kcal: 240, Protein: 4.6g, Carbs: 76g, Fats: 1.6g

45.   Sweet Artichoke Juice

Ingredients:

1 large artichoke

1 large green apple, cored

1 cup of mustard greens, torn

1 large honeydew melon wedge

1 cup of watercress, torn

2 oz of water

¼ tsp of agave nectar

Preparation:

Trim off the outer leaves of the artichoke using a sharp knife. Cut into bite-sized pieces and set aside.

Wash the apple and remove the core. Cut into bite-sized pieces and set aside.

Cut the honeydew melon lengthwise in half. Scoop out the seeds using a spoon. Cut one large wedge and peel it. Cut into small chunks and place in a bowl. Wrap the rest of the melon in a plastic foil and refrigerate.

Combine watercress and mustard greens in a colander and wash under cold running water. Drain and set aside.

Now, process artichoke, apple, honeydew melon, watercress, and mustard greens in a juicer. Transfer to serving glasses and stir in the water and agave nectar.

Add some ice and serve immediately.

Nutritional information per serving: Kcal: 261, Protein: 9.4g, Carbs: 79.6g, Fats: 1.1g

46.   Guava Melon Juice

Ingredients:

1 large guava

1 cup of watermelon

1 large orange

1 large kiwi

1 large green apple, cored

3 oz of coconut water

Preparation:

Wash the guava and cut into chunks. If you are using large fruit, reserve the rest for some other recipe in a refrigerator.

Cut the watermelon lengthwise. For one cup, you will need about one large wedge. Peel and cut into chunks. Remove the seeds and set aside. Reserve the rest of the melon for some other juices.

Peel the orange and divide into wedges. Set aside.

Peel the kiwi and cut lengthwise in half. Set aside.

Wash the apple and remove the core. Cut into bite-sized pieces and set aside.

Now, combine guava, watermelon, orange, kiwi, and apple in a juicer and process until juiced. Transfer to serving glasses and stir in the coconut water.

Add some ice or refrigerate before serving.

Enjoy!

Nutritional information per serving: Kcal: 264, Protein: 5.6g, Carbs: 73.8g, Fats: 1.6g

47.   Cherry Blueberry Juice

Ingredients:

1 cup of cherries, pitted

1 large green apple, cored

1 cup of blueberries

1 medium-sized orange

3 oz of coconut water

1 tbsp of agave nectar

Preparation:

Combine cherries and blueberries in a colander. Wash under cold running water. Drain and set aside.

Wash the apple and remove the core. Cut into bite-sized pieces and set aside.

Peel the orange and divide into wedges. Set aside.

Now, combine cherries, blueberries, apple, and orange in a juicer and process until juiced. Transfer to serving glasses and stir in the coconut water.

Add few ice cubes and serve immediately.

Enjoy!

Nutritional information per serving: Kcal: 375, Protein: 4.8g, Carbs: 91.5g, Fats: 1.3g

48.   Fennel Rosemary Juice

Ingredients:

1 large fennel

1 large Granny Smith apple

1 large cucumber

1 rosemary sprig

¼ tsp of Himalayan salt

2 oz of water

Preparation:

Wash the fennel bulb and trim off the wilted outer layers. Cut into small chunks and set aside.

Wash the apple and remove the core. Cut into bite-sized pieces and set aside.

Wash the cucumber and cut into thick pieces. Set aside.

Now, process fennel, apple, and cucumber in a juicer. Transfer to serving glasses and stir in the Himalayan salt and water. Sprinkle with rosemary and refrigerate for 30 minutes before serving.

Enjoy!

Nutritional information per serving: Kcal: 179, Protein: 5.7g, Carbs: 56g, Fats: 1.2g

49.   Strawberry Orange Juice

Ingredients:

1 cup of strawberries

1 large orange

1 cup of cantaloupe

1 large carrot

2 oz of water

Preparation:

Wash the strawberries under cold running water. Drain and cut in half. Set aside.

Peel the orange and divide into wedges. Set aside.

Cut the cantaloupe in half. Scoop out the seeds. Cut two wedges and peel them. Chop into chunks and set aside. Reserve the rest of the cantaloupe in a refrigerator.

Wash the carrot and cut into thick slices. Set aside.

Now, combine strawberries, orange, cantaloupe, and carrot in a juicer and process until juiced.

Transfer to serving glasses and stir in the water. Add some ice and serve immediately.

Nutritional information per serving: Kcal: 177, Protein: 4.9g, Carbs: 55g, Fats: 1.2g

50. Orange Cauliflower Juice

Ingredients:

1 cup of cauliflower, chopped

1 large orange

1 large carrot

1 large red bell pepper

1 cup of fresh kale, torn

¼ tsp of Himalayan salt

3 oz of water

Preparation:

Trim off the outer leaves of a cauliflower. Wash it and cut into small pieces and fill the measuring cup. Reserve the rest in the refrigerator.

Peel the orange and divide into wedges. Set aside.

Wash the carrot and cut into thick slices. Set aside.

Wash the red bell pepper and cut in half. Remove the seeds and cut in small pieces. Set aside.

Wash the kale thoroughly and torn with hands. Set aside.

Now, process cauliflower, orange, carrot, red bell pepper, and kale in a juicer. Transfer to serving glasses and stir in the salt and water.

Refrigerate for 10 minutes before serving.

Enjoy!

Nutritional information per serving: Kcal: 169, Protein: 8.9g, Carbs: 49.6g, Fats: 1.8g

51.   Plum Tomato Juice

Ingredients:

5 plum tomatoes, halved

1 cup of watercress, torn

1 cup of basil, torn

1 large green bell pepper

1 large cucumber

A handful of spinach

Preparation:

Wash the plum tomatoes and place them in a bowl. Cut in half and reserve the juice while cutting. Set aside.

Combine watercress, basil, and spinach in a colander. Wash thoroughly under cold running water. Drain and torn with hands. Set aside.

Wash the green bell pepper and cut in half. Remove the seeds and chop into small pieces. Set aside.

Wash the cucumber and cut into thick slices. Set aside.

Now, process plum tomatoes, watercress, basil, spinach, green bell pepper, and cucumber in a juicer. Transfer to serving glasses and stir in the salt and water.

Add some ice and serve.

Nutritional information per serving: Kcal: 112, Protein: 8.5g, Carbs: 32.7g, Fats: 1.5g

52.   Zucchini Beet Juice

Ingredients:

1 large zucchini

1 cup of beets, trimmed

1 large green apple

1 large radish, trimmed

1 large celery stalk, chopped

2 oz of water

Preparation:

Peel the zucchini and cut in half. Scoop out the seeds and cut into small chunks. Set aside.

Wash the beets and radish. Trim off the green parts and cut into small pieces. Set aside.

Wash the apple and remove the core. Cut into bite-sized pieces and set aside.

Wash the celery and chop it into bite-sized pieces. Set aside.

Now, combine zucchini, beets, apple, radish, and celery in a juicer and process until juiced. Transfer to serving glasses and stir in the water.

Add few ice cubes before serving and enjoy!

Nutritional information per serving: Kcal: 170, Protein: 7.3g, Carbs: 47.9g, Fats: 1.7g

53.   Cinnamon Pumpkin Juice

Ingredients:

1 cup of pumpkin chunks

1 large yellow apple, cored

1 large carrot

1 large orange

¼ tsp of cinnamon, ground

3 oz of water

Preparation:

Peel the pumpkin and cut in half. Scoop out the seeds using a spoon. Cut one large wedge and peel it. Cut into small chunks and set aside. Reserve the rest for later.

Wash the carrot and cut into thick slices. Set aside.

Wash the apple and remove the core. Cut into bite-sized pieces and set aside.

Peel the orange and divide into wedges. Set aside.

Now, process pumpkin, apple, carrot, and orange in a juicer. Transfer to serving glasses and stir in the cinnamon and water.

Add few ice cubes and serve immediately.

Enjoy!

Nutritional information per serving: Kcal: 220, Protein: 4.1g, Carbs: 65.3g, Fats: 0.8g

54.   Brussels Sprout Crookneck Squash Juice

Ingredients:

1 cup of Brussels sprouts

1 cup of crookneck squash

1 large cucumber

2 large kiwis

1 large lime

3 oz water

1 tbsp of honey

Preparation:

Wash the Brussels sprouts and trim off the outer layers. Cut in half and set aside.

Wash the crookneck squash and cut in half. Scoop out the seeds using a spoon. Cut into small chunks and fill the measuring cup. Reserve the rest for another juice.

Wash the cucumber and cut into thick slices. Set aside.

Peel the kiwis and lime. Cut lengthwise in half and set aside.

Now, combine Brussels sprouts, crookneck squash, cucumber, kiwis, and lime in a juicer and process until juiced.

Transfer to serving glasses and stir in the water and honey. Add some ice or refrigerate for 15 minutes before serving.

Enjoy!

Nutritional information per serving: Kcal: 221, Protein: 7.8g, Carbs: 64.6g, Fats: 1.7g

55. Ginger Artichoke Juice

Ingredients:

1 large artichoke

1 large grapefruit

1 large honeydew melon wedge

2 large carrots

1 small ginger root knob, 1-inch

2 oz of water

Preparation:

Using a sharp knife, trim off the outer wilted layers of artichoke. Cut into small chunks and set aside.

Peel the grapefruit and divide into wedges. Set aside.

Cut the honeydew melon lengthwise in half. Scoop out the seeds using a spoon. Cut a large wedge and peel it. Cut into small chunks and place in a bowl. Wrap the rest of the melon in a plastic foil and refrigerate.

Wash the carrots and cut into thick slices. Set aside.

Peel the ginger knob and set aside.

Now, process, artichoke, grapefruit, honeydew melon, carrots, and ginger in a juicer.

Transfer to serving glasses and stir in the water. Add some ice and serve immediately.

Enjoy!

Nutritional information per serving: Kcal: 230, Protein: 9.5g, Carbs: 72.6g, Fats: 1.1g

56. Blueberry Strawberry Juice

Ingredients:

1 cup of blueberries

1 cup of strawberries

1 medium-sized green apple, cored

1 large lemon

1 large cucumber

Preparation:

Combine blueberries and strawberries in a colander. Wash under cold running water. Drain and set aside.

Wash the apple and remove the core. Cut into bite-sized pieces and set aside.

Peel the lemon and cut lengthwise in half. set aside.

Wash the cucumber and cut into thick slices. set aside.

Now, combine blueberries, strawberries, apple, lemon, and cucumber in a juicer and process until juiced. Transfer to serving glasses and add some ice before serving.

Enjoy!

Nutritional information per serving: Kcal: 284, Protein: 6.8, Carbs: 87.9g, Fats: 2.4g

ADDITIONAL TITLES FROM THIS AUTHOR

70 Effective Meal Recipes to Prevent and Solve Being Overweight: Burn Fat Fast by Using Proper Dieting and Smart Nutrition

By

Joe Correa CSN

48 Acne Solving Meal Recipes: The Fast and Natural Path to Fixing Your Acne Problems in Less Than 10 Days!

By

Joe Correa CSN

41 Alzheimer's Preventing Meal Recipes: Reduce or Eliminate Your Alzheimer's Condition in 30 Days or Less!

By

Joe Correa CSN

70 Effective Breast Cancer Meal Recipes: Prevent and Fight Breast Cancer with Smart Nutrition and Powerful Foods

By

Joe Correa CSN